Keto Vegetarian Diet Cookbook

Ketogenic Plant Based Diet to Lose Weight Easily and Never Let It Back

By James C. Dell

Contents

Introduction

Hello friend, this is James Press! At first, I would like to congratulate you and thank you for choosing this book: "Keto Vegetarian Diet Cookbook- Ketogenic Plant Based Diet to Lose Weight Easily and Never Let It Back"

Do you want to stop the foods that go straight to your fat areas like your bum, belly, and thighs? Do you want to be slimmer or stronger than before? D**o you want to kick off all the unuseful fat and never let it come back?** What if I told you that you could lose weight fast, feel better, look more beautiful or handsome, have more energy, less pain, boost your sex drive, reduce your risk of disease… and most importantly you will still be able to eat your favorite foods? **Ketogenic Vegetarian is your answer.**

This book suits for any body weight or body shape! We have helped many people lose their weight and have a better lifestyle. We've written all that we know about ketogenic vegetarian diet, you will find essential knowledge by reading this book! You will know the basic knowledge of the ketogenic diet and its benefits, Vegetarian Diet and it's benefits. You will understand how the ketogenic vegetarian can reduce your weight faster. Meantime you will find foods that suit for ketogenic vegetarian diet and some foods that you must avoid.

So what benefits will you get by following Ketogenic Vegetarian Diet?

1. **Better skin, look younger**

2. **Rapid fat loss without exercise**

4. **Sleep better and wake up easier**

5. **Increase body energy level**

6. **Reduce the frequency of epileptic seizures**

7. **Much much more...**

This amazing fat destroying method will give you a complete body makeover without any supplements, workouts, or high-priced ineffective fat loss pills. It can work on anybody, no matter what weight, body shape, and body type you are. **You will see amazing results when you stand before the mirror in just a few weeks.**

This book is undoubtedly a must-have for those who want to know all about Ketogenic vegetarian diet. It is beautifully illustrated with 50 recipes that are keto approved, vegetarian, and over the top, scrumptious that will make anyone fall in love with this healthy diet. With a heart full of warm wishes, I welcome you to the world of the Ketogenic Vegetarian For Rapid Weight Loss.

Chapter 1: Essentials of Keto Vegetarian Diet

A Quick Overview of the Ketogenic Diet

Ketogenic Diet is getting a lot of hype these days. The word "Keto" is derived from a specific metabolic process of our body called Ketosis, our body produces Ketones.

The main aim of the Keto diet is to lower the levels of carbohydrate intake in the body while increasing the intake of fat. That is why the Keto Diet is largely known as the High-Fat Low Carb Diet or simply the Low Carb Diet. In this book, we are going to call it the "Keto Diet / Ketogenic Diet" for the sake of simplicity.

To understand how it works, we must first understand the mechanism behind it. Whenever our body is exposed to large levels of carbohydrates, the production of glucose and insulin tends to rise.

You must appreciate at this point that glucose is a very easily convertible molecule that helps the body get its energy for day to day activities. Insulin acts as a companion molecule which helps to regulate the level of glucose in our bloodstream. If glucose levels rise beyond normal, insulin helps to lower it back down. Given the fact that the body uses glucose as its core source of energy, the fat usually is not used up and stays stored inside our body.

As long as you are on a high carbohydrate diet, the fat levels won't come down because the body is always breaking down the carbohydrates first. That's why when you have a high carb diet, you must be overweight!

This is where the Ketogenic Diet kicks in. When you are depriving your body of carbohydrate, it will automatically go into a phase known as "ketosis." Here it will release a good number of Ketones that will encourage the body to take down body fat in order to supply the body with its energy. Since fat is usually present in abundance in our body, the body will have plenty of energy.

Benefits of the Ketogenic diet

Weight Loss

The first and foremost benefit of the ketogenic diet is it helps you lose weight. It does not require you to count each calorie. But it still reduces 3.2% more weight than other diet plans. Weight loss becomes essential as less carbs are used in this diet.

Reduces Hunger

Perhaps the worst side effect of dieting is hunger. It is a major flaw with dieting and discourages dieters from using their plan. However, people feel full when they are on the ketogenic diet. As fats intake increases, it keeps a person feeling satiated longer. It also helps reduce your appetite in a good way. So, it is an ideal diet for people who struggle with food cravings. It also helps reduce sugar cravings.

Fights Cancer

Cancer cells develop with sugar use. Ketogenic diet removes glucose as their primary fuel and stops taking in high carbohydrates, replacing them with fats which pushes the body's metabolism into a form or condition called ketosis. This process helps prevent and fights cancer.

Lower Blood Pressure

A low carb ketogenic diet helps lower your blood pressure. However, if you are on certain medicines, it can lead to dizziness. Check with your doctor first before going on a ketogenic diet to make sure it won't interfere with your prescriptions.

Cholesterol Killer

Cholesterol is formed when the body gets excess glucose. But when you are on a ketogenic diet, you take less sugar, and as a result, your Cholesterol reduces. Also, there is less need to repair the issues created by inflammatory chemicals.

More Energy

As keto ingredients involve more fats, it therefore, provides more energy to be active all day long. You feel full, happy, and aware all day. There is no dizziness, no low blood pressure issues, or sinking feeling. In the Indo-Pak subcontinent, people take heavy (ketogenic breakfast) by eating ghee or butter-laden flat breads called "*Parathas*with curry or spicy eggs and tea. Men eat 2 to 3 "*parathas*" in particular and do not feel any lack of energy all day long.

Helps Brain Disorders

Glucose is crucial to brain health. The brain burns it to carry out some of its most essential functions. The Ketogenic diet was basically introduced to help cure epilepsy in children. Not only has it helped with epilepsy, but it has also helped in the treatment of Parkinson's and Alzheimer's disease.

What is Vegetarian?

Traditionally, it refers to an individual who doesn't consume anything that has been slaughtered or caught. This includes every type of meat and seafood.

The Benefits Of a Vegetarian Diet

A vegetarian diet offers several advantages, below are some of them:

1. Lowers your risk of getting cancer – Studies of cancer and nutrition have shown that vegetarians are at a lower risk of contracting cancer compared to people who eat meat regularly.

2. Lose weight –According to research by the Cancer Research Center of America, people who eat meat gain more weight in a 5 year period compared to people who are vegetarians.

3. Lower your cholesterol levels – We all know eating red meat will increases our cholesterol levels. The lastest research by scientists in the USA have found that eating more plant foods will decrease cholesterol level.

4. Live longer – by following a vegetarian diet it can protect you from all kinds of diseases & ailments like cardiovascular diseases, diabetes, etc. Researchers have shown that vegetarians tend to live longer than those who eat too much meat.

In a word, the ketogenic diet restricts your carb intake, have proper proteins, and increases fat intake. The daily food intake breakdown is 10% carbs, 20% protein, and 70% fats. The Ketogenic vegetarian diet is geared towards limited and healthier proteins by restricting animal proteins. This concept further helps fighting with certain neurological conditions. By this ketogenic vegetarian diet, you will lose fat more rapidly and more healthier than other diets.

How to Lose Weight Faster Than Ever Before?

When it comes to losing weight, no diet works wonders if you're not persistent or don't loyally follow the rules. Yes, that's right! Persistency in any diet leads to success and brings you back to your ideal shape. The following are some helpful tips and tricks to help you make this diet a real success in your life.

- First and foremost clean your pantry of unhealthy and processed foods, sugars, and fast food.
- Stock your pantry with healthy and keto-friendly foods.

- Drink plenty of water.
- Grocery shop on the weekends so you can prepare your healthy keto-recipes for the upcoming week.
- Stock healthy snacks such as nuts or fresh fruits and vegetables so you don't cheat when you crave in-between meals.
- Light exercise or walking will also help you to lose weight faster.

Where Will the Ketogenic Vegetarian Diet Lead You to?

The ketogenic vegetarian diet, when followed consistently, leads you to a healthier and more energetic lifestyle. It helps you to lose weight because the stored fat is used by ketosis. Cutting out carbs lowers your glucose level and helps in reversing type 2 diabetes. The Ketosis process makes the brain use fat as a source of energy instead of using glucose which increases mental focus. It also provides higher levels of energy with increased physical endurance. Moreover, it normalizes blood pressure and helps to control epilepsy. In the long run, it can help reduce your risk of heart attack, heart diseases, cancer, Alzheimer's disease, and other such chronic diseases. A healthy diet shows on your face. You get fresher, clearer, and acne free skin. Ketogenic Vegetarian diet calms your stomach and leads you to crave less for sugars. So no more hungry feeling.

Super Tips When You Are on a Keto Vegetarian Diet

- Avoid starchy foods such as wheat, bulger, potatoes, pasta, bread, rice, or anything containing too many carbs.
- Since this diet restricts carbs you have to limit processed sugar consumption too.
- Eliminate meat from your diet.
- Don't buy restricted foods so you don't accidently cheat when on ketogenic vegetarian diet.
- You can go for healthy snacking when you crave in-between meals. Healthy snacks include nuts, seeds, fruits, or vegetables.
- Planning is very important for any diet. So better plan and shop over the weekend for the coming week meals.
- Most importantly learn to say "No" to the friends who offer you something you can't have on this diet.

Foods to Restrict in Ketogenic Vegetarian Diet

Reduce all carby foods such as wheat, bulger, potatoes, or anything containing high carbs. Since this diet restricts carbs you have to limit processed sugar consumption as well. Being vegetarian, you will also have to cut out meat.

Foods to Increase in Ketogenic Vegetarian Diet

When you restrict carbs, you have to increase healthy fat consumption such as olive oil, coconut oil, butter, nuts, avocado and seeds. Nuts and seeds will replace proteins that come from meat. Take healthy vegetables like kale, chard, spinach, broccoli, cabbage, cauliflower, and so on.

Chapter 2: Healthy & Delicious Breakfast Recipes

Simplest-Ever Spiral Veggie Salad

(Prepping time: 20 minutes| For 2 servings)

A fresh from-your-garden salad… This salad is a combo of carrot, cucumber, and kale. It is really fun to make veggie noodles with a spiral slicer.

Ingredients:

1 medium cucumber, spiralized with blade C
1 medium carrot, peeled and spiralized with blade C
1 cup of fresh baby kale, trimmed and torn
¼ cup of fresh mint leaves, chopped
2 teaspoons of balsamic vinegar
1 tablespoon of extra-virgin olive oil
Salt and freshly ground black pepper, to taste
¼ cup of walnuts, chopped

Preparation:

1. In a large serving bowl, add all ingredients except walnuts and toss to coat well.
2. Top with walnuts and serve.

Nutrition Values (per serving)

Calories: 214

Fats: 16.5g

Carbs: 14.5g

Protein: 6.4g

Fiber: 3.8g

Hot Orange Sauce with Broccoli Noodles

(Prepping time: 15 minutes| Cooking time: 12 minutes| For 4 servings)

A delicious combo of spicy and tangy flavors… Broccoli noodles are packed with the flavor of fragrant orange sauce.

Ingredients:

3 large heads of broccoli, floret and stems separated
2 tablespoons of olive oil
4 garlic cloves, minced
¼ teaspoon of red pepper flakes, crushed
Salt and freshly ground black pepper, to taste
1/3 cup of fresh orange juice
1 teaspoon of fresh orange zest, grated finely

Preparation:

1. With the B blade of the vegetable spiralizer, make noodles out of the broccoli stems.

2. In a large pot of lightly salted boiling water, add broccoli noodles and florets and cook for about 2-3 minutes.

3. Drain well and with a paper towel, pat dry the florets and noodles.

4. In a large skillet, heat oil over medium heat.

5. Add the garlic and red pepper flakes and sauté for about 1 minute.

6. Add the broccoli florets and noodles and cook, covered for about 2-3 minutes.

7. Add remaining ingredients and cook for about 5 minutes, stirring occasionally.

8. Serve hot.

Nutrition Values (per serving)

Calories: 146

Fats: 7.8g

Carbs: 17.3g

Protein: 6.2g

Fiber: 5.6g

Magnificent Barbecue Flavored Zucchini Noodles

(Prepping time: 15 minutes| Cooking time: 12 minutes| For 4 servings)

A heavenly tasty and perfectly healthy zucchini plate… Fresh zucchini noodles are mixed with a delicious barbecue sauce.

Ingredients:

- 2 tablespoons of olive oil
- 2 yellow onions, sliced thinly
- 4 small zucchinis, spiralized with blade C
- ¼ cup of sugar-free barbecue sauce (of your choice)

Preparation:

1. In a large skillet, heat oil over medium heat.

2. Add the onions and sauté for about 4-5 minutes.

3. Add the zucchini noodles and cook for about 2 minutes.

4. Stir in the barbecue sauce and cook for about 3-5 minutes or till desired doneness.

5. Serve hot.

Nutrition Values (per serving)

Calories: 124

Fats: 7.3g

Carbs: 14.8g

Protein: 2g

Fiber: 2.6g

Tasty Cauliflower Noodles with Protein-Rich Tofu

(Prepping time: 15 minutes| Cooking time: 10 minutes| For 4 servings)

One of the heartier and protein-rich meals…Cauliflower noodles are combined with protein-rich tofu with a nice balsamic ginger sauce.

Ingredients:

2 medium heads of cauliflower, floret and stems separated
3 tablespoons of coconut aminos
3½ tablespoons of olive oil, divided (1 ½ tablespoosn & 2 tablespoons)
½ teaspoon of balsamic vinegar
1 pound of extra-firm tofu, drained and cubed
½ tablespoon of fresh ginger, grated finely
Salt and freshly ground black pepper, to taste

Preparation:

1. In a bowl, mix together the coconut aminos, 1½ tablespoons of oil, and vinegar. Set aside.

2. With the B blade of a vegetable spiralizer, make noodles out of the cauliflower stems.

3. In a large pan of lightly salted boiling water, add broccoli noodles and florets and cook for about 4-5 minutes.

4. Drain well and with a paper towel, pat dry the noodles.

5. Transfer the cauliflower noodles into a large bowl.

6. Add half of coconut aminos mixture and toss to coat well.

7. In a large skillet, heat remaining oil on medium heat.

8. Add tofu and cook for about 2-3 minutes per side.

9. Add remaining coconut aminos mixture and ginger and cook for about 1-2 minute.

10. Season with desired amount of salt and black pepper.

11. Divide cauliflower noodles on serving plates.

12. Top with tofu and serve.

Nutrition Values (per serving)

Calories: 291

Fats: 19.2g

Carbs: 19.2g

Protein: 17.8g

Fiber: 8g

Baked Tofu Delight with Pumpkin Noodles

(Prepping time: 15 minutes| Cooking time: 30 minutes| For 4 servings)

A unique combination of baked tofu and stir fried pumpkin noodles… Baking gives the tofu a perfect texture with a nice glazed coating of subtle flavors.

Ingredients:

For Tofu:

> 1/3 cup of coconut Aminos
> 2 tablespoons of balsamic vinegar
> ½ tablespoon of garlic, minced
> 1 (16-ounce) package of extra-firm tofu, drained and cubed
> ½ tablespoon of olive oil

For Pumpkin Noodles:

> 1 tablespoon of olive oil
> 2 garlic cloves, minced
> ¼ teaspoon of red pepper flakes, crushed
> 3 cups of pumpkins, peeled spiralized with blade C
> Salt and freshly ground black pepper, to taste

Preparation:

1. For tofu, in a bowl, mix together coconut aminos, vinegar, and garlic.

2. Add tofu cubes and coat with mixture generously.

3. Refrigerate, covered for about 5 hours.

4. Preheat the oven to 400 degrees F. Grease a baking sheet.

5. Remove tofu from marinade and arrange onto prepared baking sheet leaving space in between each cube.

6. Bake for about 15 minutes per side.

7. Meanwhile, for pumpkin noodles, in a big skillet, heat oil on medium heat.

8. Add garlic and red pepper flakes and sauté for about 1 minute.

9. Add pumpkin noodles and cook for about 4-5 minutes.

10. Season with salt and black pepper and remove from heat.

11. Divide pumpkin noodles on serving plates.

12. Top with tofu and serve.

Nutrition Values (per serving)

Calories: 228

Fats: 12.4g

Carbs: 19.7g

Protein: 14.8g

Fiber: 6g

Sweet & Spicy Carrot Noodles

(Prepping time: 15 minutes| Cooking time: 12 minutes| For 4 servings)

One of the easiest and best ways to enjoy a healthy carrot in a delish way… These delicious and totally healthy carrot noodles are covered in a sweet, tangy, and spicy sauce.

Ingredients:

2 tablespoons of olive oil
¼ cup of white onion, chopped
2 garlic cloves, minced
2 Serrano peppers, seeded and chopped
3 large carrots, peeled and spiralized with blade C
2 tablespoons of fresh lime juice
8-10 drops of liquid stevia
Salt and freshly ground black pepper, to taste
¼ cup of scallions, chopped

Preparation:

1. In a large skillet, heat oil on medium heat.

2. Add onion and sauté for about 4-5 minutes.

3. Add garlic and Serrano peppers and sauté for 1 minute.

4. Add carrots and sauté for about 4-5 minutes.

5. Stir in stevia, lime juice, salt, and black pepper and cook for about 1 minute.

6. Remove from heat and serve immediately, garnishing of scallion.

Nutrition Values (per serving)

Calories: 92

Fats: 7g

Carbs: 7.8g

Protein: 0.8g

Fiber: 1.8g

Bright Green Noodles with Exotic Mushroom Sauce

(Prepping time: 20 minutes| Cooking time: 12 minutes| For 4 servings)

A wonderful recipe of zucchini noodles and creamy mushroom sauce…This creamy mushroom sauce is really packed with rich flavors.

Ingredients:

For Mushroom Sauce:

> 1½ tablespoons of olive oil
> 1 garlic clove, minced
> 1¼ cups of fresh button mushrooms, sliced
> ¼ cup of vegetable broth
> ¼ cup of sour cream
> Salt and freshly ground black pepper, to taste

For Green Noodles:

> 3 large zucchinis, spiralized with blade C
> ¼ cup of fresh parsley, chopped

Preparation:

1. In a large skillet, heat oil on medium heat.

2. Add garlic and sauté for about 1 minute.

3. Add mushrooms and cook 6-8 minutes.

4. Add broth and cook for about 2 minutes, stirring continuously.

5. Stir in sour cream, salt, and black pepper and cook for about 1 minute.

6. Remove from heat.

7. Meanwhile, cook noodles in a pan of boiling water, add zucchini and cook for about 2-3 minutes.

8. With a slotted spoon, transfer zucchini noodles into a colander and immediately run cold water over them.

9. Drain well and transfer the zucchini noodles on a large plate lined with paper towel. Pat noodles dry.

10. Now, divide the zucchini noodles onto serving plates.

11. Top with mushroom sauce evenly.

12. Garnish with the parsley and serve.

Nutrition Values (per serving)

Calories: 124

Fats: 8.9g

Carbs: 10g

Protein: 4.5g

Fiber: 3g

Majestic Hot & Sour Pumpkin Soupy Noodles

(Prepping time: 15 minutes| Cooking time: 20 minutes| For 4 servings)

A flavorful soup with a delicious and hot and spicy kick… Pumpkin noodles in hot soup give a luxurious bite to this delicious soup. Garnishing of fresh basil adds an aromatic touch in the soup.

Ingredients:

2 tablespoons of olive oil
1 medium onion, chopped
1 garlic clove, minced
2 Serrano peppers, seeded and chopped finely
1 teaspoon of ground cumin
1 teaspoon of red pPepper flakes, crushed
1 cup of tomatoes, chopped finely
4 cups of vegetable broth
3 tablespoons fresh lemon juice
2 cups of pumpkin, peeled and spiralized with blade C
Salt and freshly ground black pepper, to taste
2 tablespoons of fresh basil leaves, chopped

Preparation:

1. In a large soup pan, heat oil on medium heat.

2. Add onion and sauté for about 4-5 minutes.

3. Add garlic, Serrano peppers, cumin, and red pepper flakes and sauté for about 1 minute.

4. Add tomatoes and cook for about 2-3 minutes, crushing with the back of a spoon.

5. Add broth and lemon juice and bring to a boil.

6. Cook for about 2-3 minutes.

7. Stir in pumpkin noodles and reduce the heat to medium-low.

8. Simmer for about 6-8 minutes.

9. Stir in salt and black pepper and immediately remove from heat.

10. Garnish with basil and serve.

<u>Nutrition Values (per serving)</u>

Calories: 168

Fats: 9.1g

Carbs: 16.4g

Protein: 7.3g

Fiber: 5.1g

Carrot Noodles with Baked Tofu & Lemony Yogurt Sauce

(Prepping time: 20 minutes| Cooking time: 1 hour | For 4 servings)

A combination of carrots, tofu, and yogurt sauce… This recipe prepares a really healthy platter of nutritious ingredients like carrots and tofu with refreshing lemony yogurt sauce…

Ingredients:

For Tofu:

- 1 teaspoon of fresh ginger, minced
- 1 teaspoon of garlic, minced
- 2 tablespoons of coconut aminos
- 1 tablespoon of olive oil
- 1 pound of tofu, drained and cut into 8 slices

For Yogurt Sauce:

- ½ cup of plain greek yogurt
- 2 tablespoons of chives, minced
- 2 teaspoons of fresh lemon zest, grated finely
- 2 teaspoons of fresh lemon juice
- Salt, to taste

For Carrot Noodles:

- 2 large carrots, peeled and spiralized with blade C
- 1½ tablespoon of olive oil

Preparation:

1. Preheat the oven to 350 degrees F. Lightly, grease a baking sheet.

2. In a bowl, mix together all ingredients except tofu.

3. Coat the tofu with half of ginger mixture evenly.

4. Arrange the tofu cubes onto prepared baking sheet in a single layer.

5. Bake for about 30 minutes.

6. Flip the tofu slices and coat with remaining ginger mixture evenly.

7. Bake for about 30 minutes.

8. Meanwhile, in a bowl, add all the ingredients for the yogurt sauce and stir to combine well.

9. In a large bowl, add carrot noodles and oil and toss to coat well.

10. Divide carrot noodles on 4 serving plates evenly.

11. Place 2 tofu slices on each plate.

12. Top with yogurt sauce evenly and serve.

Nutrition Values (per serving)

Calories: 201

Fats: 14.2g

Carbs: 8.2g

Protein: 13.4g

Fiber: 2.1g

Colorful Vegetable Salad with Feta Cheese

(Prepping time: 20 minutes| For 4 servings)

A bowl of garden fresh veggie noodles that looks like a beautiful rainbow… This salad bowl is bursting with the flavors of freshness. Surely this salad will be a hit for friends and family gathering.

Ingredients:

For Salad:

2 medium beets, trimmed, peeled and spiralized with blade C
1 large carrot, peeled and spiralized with blade C
1 large zucchini, spiralized with blade C
1 large cucumber, spiralized with blade C
¼ cup of feta cheese, crumbled

For Dressing:

1 garlic clove, minced
¼ cup of fresh cilantro, minced
¼ cup of apple cider vinegar
¼ cup of extra-virgin olive oil
Salt and freshly ground black pepper, to taste

Preparation:

1. In a large serving bowl, add all salad ingredients except the cheese.

2. In another bowl, add all dressing ingredients and beat until well combined.

3. Pour dressing over salad and toss to coat well.

4. Top with cheese and serve.

Nutrition Values (per serving)

Calories: 187

Fats: 14.9g

Carbs: 12.1g

Protein: 3.7g

Fiber: 2.6g

Spring Onion Omelet

(Prepping time: 10 minutes| Cooking time: 4 minutes| For 2 servings)

One of the easiest and delicious cheese and spring onion stuffed omelet for a nice winter morning breakfast…. Of course this omelet is healthy as well.

Ingredients:

4 organic Eggs
3 tablespoons of milk
½ cup of spring onions, chopped finely
2 tablespoons of cheddar cheese, grated
¼ teaspoon of red pepper flakes, crushed
Salt and freshly ground black pepper, to taste
2 teaspoons of butter

Preparation:

1. In a bowl, add eggs and milk and beat well.

2. Add remaining ingredients except butter and mix well.

3. In a large frying pan, melt butter on medium heat.

4. Add egg mixture and with a spatula, spread in the bottom of the pan.

5. Reduce the heat to low and cook for about 2 minutes.

6. Fold the omelet and cook for about 1-2 minutes or until egs are set completely.

Nutrition Values (per serving)

Calories: 208

Fats: 15.5g

Carbs: 3.9g

Protein: 14.1g

Fiber: 0.7g

Sweet Cashew & Raspberry Smoothie

(Prepping time: 10 minutes| For 2 servings)

A sweet smoothie that is made with sweet raspberries and healthy cashews… The cashews give a delightful creamy base to this smoothie.

Ingredients:

¾ cup of frozen raspberries
1 teaspoon of cashews
2-3 drops of liquid stevia
1½ cups of unsweetened coconut milk

Preparation:

1. In a high speed blender, add all ingredients and pulse till smooth.
2. Pour into 2 serving glasses and serve immediately.

Nutrition Values (per serving)

Calories: 135

Fats: 3.4g

Carbs: 26.5g

Protein: 1.6g

Fiber: 4.9g

Warm Strawberry Coconut Flakes

(Prepping time: 10 minutes| Cooking time: 30 minutes| For 4 servings)

A wholesome and fruity porridge that will warm you in a nice way…Lemon juice adds a refreshingly tasty touch into this porridge.

Ingredients:

> 1 pound of fresh strawberries, hulled and sliced
> 1 tablespoon of fresh lemon juice
> 8-10 drops of liquid stevia
> ¼ cup of water
> 1/3 cup of unsweetened coconut flakes

Preparation:

1. In a medium pot, add all ingredients on medium heat and bring to a boil.

2. Reduce the heat to medium-low and simmer for about 20-30 minutes, stirring occasionally.

3. Remove from heat and keep aside to cool slightly.

4. Serve warm with the topping of coconut flakes.

Nutrition Values (per serving)

Calories: 61

Fats: 2.6g

Carbs: 9.8g

Protein: 1g

Fiber: 2.9g

Eggs Stuffed with Avocado & Watercress

(Prepping time: 15 minutes| Cooking time: 5 minutes| For 6 servings)

A recipe of stuffed eggs that is really easy to make and delicious as well. These stuffed eggs have a healthy and beautifully green colored twist and are also a great option for larger gatherings.

Ingredients:

6 organic eggs
1/3 cup of fresh watercress, trimmed
1 medium ripe avocado, peeled, pitted and chopped
½ tablespoon of fresh lemon juice
Salt, to taste
1/8 teaspoon of paprika

Preparation:

1. In a large pan of water, add eggs and bring to a boil on high heat.

2. Cover the pan and reduce the heat to medium-low.

3. Cook for about 4 minutes.

4. Remove from heat and keep aside, covered for about 10-12 minutes.

5. Meanwhile arrange a steamer basket over a pan of water.

6. Place the watercress in steamer basket and steam for about 1 minute.

7. Drain the watercress completely and squeeze well.

8. Remove the eggs from pan and rinse under cold water for about 1 minute.

9. Now, peel the eggs and cut in half lengthwise.

10. Remove the egg yolks and transfer into a bowl.

11. Add watercress, avocado, lemon juice, and salt and with a fork, mash completely.

12. Arrange the egg whites on a serving plate.

13. Stuff the egg whites with watercress mixture evenly.

14. Sprinkle with paprika and serve.

Nutrition Values (per serving)

Calories: 132

Fats: 10.9g

Carbs: 3.3g

Protein: 6.3g

Fiber: 2.3g

Grilled Pepper & Tomato Omelet

(Prepping time: 15 minutes| Cooking time: 20 minutes| For 4 servings)

An awesome veggie-packed omelet that is perfect for a delicious breakfast…This omelet is a flavorful blend of eggs, charred bell peppers, and juicy tomatoes. Grilled peppers add a rich flavor in this omelet.

Ingredients:

For Grilled Pepper:

> 1 large ell pepper, halved and cored
> ½ teaspoon of olive oil

For Omelet:

> 6 organic eggs
> Salt and freshly ground black pepper, to taste
> 3 tablespoons of olive oil, divided
> 1 medium onion, chopped
> 2 medium tomatoes, seeded and chopped

Preparation:

1. Preheat the grill to medium-high heat. Grease the grill grate.

2. Drizzle the bell pepper with oil.

3. Grill for about 2 minutes per side.

4. Remove from heat and keep aside to cool.

5. Then chop the bell pepper.

6. In a bowl, add eggs, salt, and black pepper and beat well.

7. In a large frying pan, heat 1½ tablespoons of oil on medium-high heat.

8. Add onion and tomatoes and sauté for about 4 minutes.

9. Add bell pepper and sauté for about 1-2 minute more.

10. Transfer the tomato mixture into a bowl.

11. In the same skillet, heat remaining oil on medium heat.

12. Add egg mixture and with a spatula, spread in the bottom evenly.

13. Cook for about 2-3 minutes.

14. Place the tomato mixture over the egg mixture and cook for about 1 minute.

15. Once the eggs are set, fold the omelet and transfer onto a serving plate.

Nutrition Values (per serving)

Calories: 221

Fats: 17.9g

Carbs: 7.7g

Protein: 9.4g

Fiber: 1.7g

Chapter 3: Mouth-Watering Lunch Recipes

Rosy Summer Cool Yogurt Shake

(Prepping time: 10 minutes| For 2 servings)

One of the most amazingly tasty shakes with a rich creamy texture... Combo of skim milk and Greek yogurt provides a creamy base. This very filling shake has a bright pink rosy color.

Ingredients:

1 cup of fresh strawberries
½ cup of plain greek yogurt
½ cup of skim milk
4-6 drops of liquid stevia
¼ cup of ice cubes

Preparation:

1. In a high speed blender, add all the ingredients and pulse till smooth.
2. Pour into 2 serving glasses and serve immediately.

Nutrition Values (per serving)

Calories: 163

Fats: 12.7g

Carbs: 6.6g

Protein: 17.1g

Fiber: 1.4g

Cinnamon Delight Yogurt Shake

(Prepping time: 10 minutes| For 2 servings)

A heart healthy and nutrient packed shake… Whip up this delicious and healthy pumpkin treat in Greek yogurt for a wonderful shake. Ground cinnamon adds a delicious and aromatic touch in this shake.

Ingredients:

¾ cup of pumpkin puree
½ cup of plain greek yogurt
1 tablespoon of ground flax seeds
½ tablespoon of ground cinnamon
½ cup of unsweetened coconut milk
4-6 drops of liquid stevia
¼ cup of ice cubes

Preparation:

1. In a high speed blender, add all the ingredients and pulse till smooth.
2. Pour into 2 serving glasses and serve immediately.

Nutrition Values (per serving)

Calories: 239

Fats: 16.9g

Carbs: 5.6g

Protein: 9.4g

Fiber: 5.8g

Triple Berry Delightful Smoothie

(Prepping time: 10 minutes| For 2 servings)

One the most delicious smoothies that is super healthy as well… This shake makes a great treat on hot summer days.

Ingredients:

> 1/3 cup of frozen strawberries
> ¼ cup of frozen blackberries
> ¼ cup of frozen blueberries
> ½ cup of fresh spinach
> 4-6 drops of liquid stevia
> 1 cup of unsweetened coconut milk

Preparation:

1. In a high speed blender, add all he ingredients and pulse till smooth.
2. Pour into 2 serving glasses and serve immediately.

Nutrition Values (per serving)

Calories: 304

Fats: 28.8g

Carbs: 13.4g

Protein: 3.4g

Fiber: 4.7g

Mango Tango Yogurt Shake

(Prepping time: 10 minutes| For 2 servings)

A pretty yellow colored shake with the flavor of sweet mango… This shake is prepared without any kind of sweetener. This creamy mango shake is a combo of sweet mango, yogurt, and almond milk.

Ingredients:

½ cup of frozen mangoes, peeled, pitted and chopped
½ cup of plain greek yogurt
½ cup of unsweetened almond milk
¼ cup of ice cubes

Preparation:

1. In a high speed blender, add all the ingredients and pulse till smooth.
2. Pour into 2 serving glasses and serve immediately.

Nutrition Values (per serving)

Calories: 142

Fats: 27g

Carbs: 15g

Protein: 7.7g

Fiber: 2.4g

Ketogenic Cabbage & Pumpkin Soup

(Prepping time: 15 minutes| Cooking time: 50 minutes| For 6 servings)

A healthy, hearty and filling soup with a light creamy texture... This soup is filled with the delish flavors of cabbage, pumpkin, coconut milk and broth. Surely this hearty and filling soup will become a family favorite.

Ingredients:

2 tablespoons of olive oil
½ cup of onion, chopped
1 teaspoon of fresh ginger, grated
2 garlic cloves, minced
1¼ cups of pumpkin, peeled and chopped
1¼ cups of cabbage, chopped
3 cups of vegetable broth
3 cups of water
1 scallion, Chopped
½ cup of fresh cilantro, chopped
½ cup of unsweetened coconut milk
Salt and freshly ground black pepper, to taste

Preparation:

1. In a large soup pan, heat oil on medium heat.

2. Add onion and sauté for about 4-5 minutes.

3. Add scallion, ginger, and garlic and sauté for about 2 minutes.

4. Add pumpkin and cabbage and cook for about 10 minutes, stirring occasionally.

5. Add broth and water and bring to a boil.

6. Reduce the heat to medium-low and simmer for about 20 minutes.

7. Stir in scallions and cilantro and simmer for about 10 minutes more.

8. Stir in coconut milk, salt, and black pepper and simmer for about 2-3 minutes.

9. Serve hot.

Nutrition Values (per serving)

Calories: 134

Fats: 10.3g

Carbs: 8.2g

Protein: 3.9g

Fiber: 2.7g

Nutty Majestic Avocado

(Prepping time: 20 minutes| Cooking time: 10 minutes| For 6 servings)

One of the most amazingly delicious recipes of stuffed avocados…Tofu, broccoli, and avocado make a perfect trio in this meal. Grilling adds a delicious smoky touch to the broccoli and tofu.

Ingredients:

For Marinade:

¼ cup of fresh cilantro leaves, chopped
1 garlic clove, minced
1 teaspoon of fresh lemon zest, grated finely
1 tablespoon of dijon mustard
¼ cup of extra-virgin olive oil
2 tablespoons of fresh lemon juice
¼ teaspoon of ground cumin
Salt and freshly ground black pepper, to taste
1 (8-ounce) package of firm tofu, drained and cut into ½-inch slices
1 cup of broccoli florets

For Stuffed Avocados:

1 tablespoon of chives, minced
3 firm avocados, halved and pitted
Salt and freshly ground black pepper, to taste
1/3 cup of sour cream

Preparation:

1. Prepare marinade in a large bowl. Add all the marinade ingredients except tofu and broccoli and beat until well combined.

2. Add tofu and broccoli and coat with marinade generously.

3. Refrigerate, covered for about 1 hour.

4. Preheat the grill to medium-high heat. Grease the grill grate.

5. Grill the tofu slices for about 2 minutes per side.

6. Grill the broccoli florets for about 8-10 minutes, flipping occasionally.

7. Remove the tofu and broccoli from the grill and chop into tiny pieces.

8. Transfer the tofu and broccoli in a bowl with chives and mix well.

9. Sprinkle the avocado halves with salt and black pepper.

10. Stuff each half with tofu mixture.

11. Top with sour cream and serve.

Nutrition Values (per serving)

Calories: 341

Fats: 32.5g

Carbs: 11.4g

Protein: 6.1g

Fiber: 7.6g

Creamy Cheese Avocado

(Prepping time: 10 minutes| For 8 servings)

A yummy and richly creamy treat of avocado… This creamy treat can be made very quickly, but is sure to impress all.

Ingredients:

1 avocado, peeled, pitted and chopped
3-ounce of cream cheese, softened
2 garlic cloves, minced
1 tablespoon of fresh lemon juice
Salt and freshly ground black pepper, to taste

Preparation:

1. In a bowl, add the avocado and with a fork, mash it completely.

2. Add remaining ingredients and stir to combine well.

3. Refrigerate before serving.

Nutrition Values (per serving)

Calories: 90

Fats: 8.6g

Carbs: 2.7g

Protein: 1.4g

Fiber: 1.7g

Portobello Mushroom Burgers

(Prepping time: 15 minutes| Cooking time: 16 minutes| For 4 servings)

An excellent recipe for a delicious lunch… Even mushroom haters will love to enjoy these burgers. A combo of herbs, garlic, balsamic vinegar, and cheese gives these mushroom caps a delightful flavoring.

Ingredients:

4 portobello mushroom caps
1 tablespoon of garlic, minced
1 teaspoon of dried oregano, crushed
1 teaspoon of dried basil, crushed
¼ cup of balsamic vinegar
2 tablespoons of Olive Oil
Salt and freshly ground black pepper, to taste
4 (1-ounce) parmesan cheese Slices

Preparation:

1. Arrange the mushroom caps in a shallow dish, smooth side up.

2. In a bowl, add remaining ingredients except cheese slices and beat until well combined.

3. Pour herb mixture over mushroom caps evenly.

4. Keep aside in room temperature for about 15-20 minutes.

5. Preheat the grill to medium-high heat. Grease the grill grate.

6. Remove the mushroom caps from dish, reserving the marinade.

7. Arrange the mushroom caps onto prepared grill grate.

8. Grill for about 5-8 minutes per side, coating with reserved marinade occasionally.

9. In the last 2 minutes of cooking, top each mushroom cap with 1 cheese slice.

Nutrition Values (per serving)

Calories: 180

Fats: 13.3g

Carbs: 6.3g

Protein: 11.4g

Fiber: 1.5g

Baked Zucchini with Blue Cheese Drizzle

(Prepping time: 15 minutes| Cooking time: 25 minutes| For 6 servings)

A sure to impress recipe of summer zucchini… Baking with blue cheese prepares a wonderful meal for the whole family. This impressive recipe needs only uses 3 ingredients to prepare such a delicious dish.

Ingredients:

6 baby zucchinis, halved lengthwise
1 tablespoon of olive oil
½ cup of blue cheese, crumbled

Preparation:

1. Preheat the oven to 450 degrees F. Arrange the rack in the center of the oven.

2. Line a baking sheet with a piece of foil.

3. Coat the zucchini halves with oil evenly.

4. Arrange the zucchini halves onto prepared baking sheet, cut side down.

5. Roast for about 15-20 minutes.

6. Remove the baking sheet from oven and sprinkle each zucchini half with cheese evenly.

7. Roast for about 3-5 minutes more.

Nutrition Values (per serving)

Calories: 91

Fats: 8.9g

Carbs: 6.8g

Protein: 4.8g

Fiber: 2.2g

Hot Chili Cauliflower Stew

(Prepping time: 15 minutes| Cooking time: 55 minutes| For 4 servings)

An excellent recipe with healthy ingredients. This vegetarian stew is chocked full of a delicious spicy kick… Cauliflower and tomatoes are the main base of this flavorful sew.

Ingredients:

2 tablespoons of olive oil
2 medium red onion, chopped
3 garlic cloves, minced
1 teaspoon of fresh ginger, minced
1 fresh green chili, seeded and chopped
½ teaspoon of dried thyme, crushed
1 teaspoon of ground cumin
½ teaspoon of cayenne pepper
2 cups of tomatoes, chopped finely
1 medium head of cauliflower, cut into florets
1 bay leaf
2 tablespoons of tomato paste
1¼ cups of vegetable broth
2 tablespoons of fresh lemon juice
Salt and freshly ground black pepper, to taste
2 tablespoons of fresh cilantro, chopped

Preparation:

1. In a Dutch oven, heat oil on medium heat.

2. Add onion and sauté for about 8-9 minutes.

3. Add garlic, ginger, chili, thyme, and remaining spices and sauté for about 1 minute.

4. Add tomatoes and cook for about 2-3 minutes, crushing with the back of spoon.

5. Add cauliflower and cook for about 2 minutes.

6. Add bay leaf, tomato paste, and broth and bring to a boil.

7. Reduce the heat to low and simmer, covered for about 30-40 minutes.

8. Stir in lemon juice, salt, and black pepper and remove from heat.

9. Garnish with cilantro and serve hot.

Nutrition Values (per serving)

Calories: 133

Fats: 8g

Carbs: 3.4g

Protein: 3.8g

Fiber: 3.2g

Zucchini Oven Baked Rings

(Prepping time: 15 minutes| Cooking time: 10 minutes| For 4 servings)

Delicious baked zucchini rings that seal in all of the fantastic natural juiciness of zucchini... The preparation method of these zucchini rings is very simple.

Ingredients:

    2 medium zucchinis, cut into ¼-inch thick rings
    2 tablespoons of extra-virgin olive oil
    1 garlic clove, minced
    1 tablespoon fresh rosemary, minced
    Salt and freshly ground black pepper, to taste
    2 tablespoons of parmesan cheese, grated

Preparation:

1. Preheat the oven to 400 degrees F. Grease a baking sheet.

2. In a bowl, add all the ingredients and toss to coat well.

3. Arrange the zucchini mixture onto prepared baking sheet in a single layer.

4. Bake for about 10 minutes, flipping once halfway through.

Nutrition Values (per serving)

Calories: 91

Fats: 8.1g

Carbs: 4.2g

Protein: 2.4g

Fiber: 1.5g

Lean Tomato Stew

(Prepping time: 15 minutes | Cooking time: 26 minutes | For 4 servings)

A great vegetarian stew that prepares an absolutely delicious meal for lunch… This stew is a delicious combination of tomatoes, celery, thyme, and spices.

Ingredients:

4 large tomatoes
2 tablespoons of olive oil
1 celery stalk, chopped finely
1 onion, chopped finely
½ teaspoon of dried thyme, crushed
¼ teaspoon of cayenne pepper
Salt and freshly ground black pepper, to taste
2 cups of water

Preparation:

1. In a pan of boiling water, soak the tomatoes for about 1 minute.

2. Drain well and gently, remove the skin.

3. In a large pan, heat oil on medium heat.

4. Add onion and celery and sauté for about 4-5 minutes.

5. Add tomatoes and remaining ingredients and bring to a boil.

6. Cook, covered for about 15-20 minutes, stirring occasionally.

7. Serve hot

Nutrition Values (per serving)

Calories: 105

Fats:9.4g

Carbs: 6g

Protein: 2g

Fiber: 2.9g

Chapter 4: Best Keto Vegetarian Dinner Recipes

Roasted Pepper & Cauliflower Soup

(Prepping time: 15 minutes| Cooking time: 1 hour 15 minutes| For 5 servings)

An outstanding vegetarian soup with the combo of a rich creamy texture and hot spicy touch… Roasting gives a delicious touch to the cauliflower and bell peppers.

Ingredients:

2 medium red bell peppers, halved and seeded
½ head of cauliflower, cut into florets
¼ cup of olive oil, divided
Salt and freshly ground black pepper, to taste
3 scallions, chopped
1 teaspoon of dried thyme, crushed
1 teaspoon of garlic powder
1 teaspoon of smoked paprika
¼ teaspoon of red pepper flakes, crushed
3 cups of vegetable broth
½ cup of heavy cream
¼ cup of fresh parsley, chopped

Preparation:

1. Preheat the broiler of oven. Line a baking sheet with a piece of foil.

2. Arrange the bell peppers onto prepared baking sheet, skin side up.

3. Broil for about 10-15 minutes.

4. Transfer the peppers into a container.

5. Cover the container tightly and keep aside while cauliflowers roasts.

6. Now, set the oven to 400 degrees F.

7. In a bowl, add cauliflower, 2 tablespoons of oil, salt, and black pepper and toss to coat well.

8. Arrange the cauliflower onto foil lined baking sheet.

9. Roast for about 30-35 minutes.

10. Remove the peppers from container.

11. Carefully, peel the skin and chop roughly.

12. In a large pan, heat remaining oil on medium heat.

13. Add scallions and sauté for about 2-3 minutes.

14. Add thyme and other spices and sauté for about 1 minute.

15. Add broth, peppers, and cauliflower and bring to a boil.

16. Reduce the heat to medium-low and simmer for about 15-20 minutes.

17. With an immerse blender, blend the mixture till smooth.

18. Stir in cream, salt, and black pepper and remove from heat.

19. Garnish with parsley and serve hot.

Nutrition Values (per serving)

Calories: 181

Fats: 15.6g

Carbs: 7.6g

Protein: 4.6g

Fiber: 1.9g

Greek-Style Creamy Spinach Pie

(Prepping time: 15 minutes| Cooking time: 50 minutes| For 8 servings)

An authentic Greek style crustless pie… This pie is stuffed with spinach, scallions, eggs, sour cream, Parmesan and feta cheeses, and fresh lemon juice. This pie will be a hit for holiday's dinners.

Ingredients:

20-ounce of frozen chopped spinach, thawed and squeezed
8 scallions, sliced
3 large organic eggs, beaten lightly
1/3 cup of low-fat sour cream
1/3 cup of parmesan cheese, grated
4-ounce of feta cheese, crumbled
2 tablespoons of fresh lemon juice
1 tablespoon of olive oil
2 teaspoons of dill weed
Salt and freshly ground black pepper, to taste

Preparation:

1. Preheat the oven to 375 degrees F. Grease a glass pie dish.

2. In a bowl, add all the ingredients and mix until well combined.

3. Transfer the mixture into the prepared pie dish evenly.

4. Bake for about 45-50 minutes or until top becomes golden brown.

Nutrition Values (per serving)

Calories: 139

Fats: 10.1g

Carbs: 5.2g

Protein: 8.7g

Fiber: 2g

Sweet Asparagus with Parmesan Cheese

(Prepping time: 10 minutes| Cooking time: 12 minutes| For 4 servings)

A perfect spring time meal of asparagus… Roasting of the asparagus brings out its natural sweetness nicely.

Ingredients:

1 pound of fresh asparagus, trimmed
1 tablespoon of olive oil
Salt and freshly ground black pepper, to taste
¼ cup of parmesan cheese, shredded

Preparation:

1. Preheat the oven to 400 degrees F. Grease a 13x9-inch casserole dish.

2. Arrange asparagus onto prepared casserole dish.

3. Drizzle with oil and sprinkle with salt and black pepper.

4. Top with cheese evenly.

5. Roast for about 12 minutes.

Nutrition Values (per serving)

Calories: 75

Fats: 7.1g

Carbs: 4.7g

Protein: 4.7g

Fiber: 2.4g

Ketogenic Cabbage Rolls

(Prepping time: 25 minutes| Cooking time: 20 minutes| For 8 servings)

Sure to bea family favorite recipe for dinner… These vegetable stuffed rolls would also be great for special occasions. Tomato sauce enhances the flavor of the cabbage rolls.

Ingredients:

For Filling:

> 1½ cups of fresh mushrooms, chopped
> 3 cups of zucchini, chopped
> 1 cup of red bell pepper, seeded and chopped
> 1 cup of green bell pepper, seeded and chopped
> ½ teaspoon of dried thyme, crushed
> ½ teaspoon of dried marjoram, crushed
> ½ teaspoon of dried basil, crushed
> Salt and freshly ground black pepper, to taste
> ¾ cup of vegetable broth
> ¼ cup of parmesan cheese, shredded
> 2 teaspoons of fresh lemon juice

For Rolls:

> 8 cabbage leaves
> 8-ounce of sugar-free tomato Sauce
> 2 tablespoons of parmesan cheese, shredded

Preparation:

1. Preheat the oven to 400 degrees F. Grease a 13x9-inch casserole dish.

2. To prepare filling, in a large pan, add all the ingredients except cheese and lemon juice on medium heat and bring to a boil.

3. Reduce the heat and simmer, covered for about 5 minutes.

4. Remove from heat and keep aside for about 5 minutes.

5. Add cheese and lemon juice and stir to combine.

6. Meanwhile in a large pan of boiling water, add cabbage leaves and boil for about 2-4 minutes.

7. Drain well.

8. In each cabbage leaf, make a V shape cut by cutting the thick vein.

9. Before filling, overlap cut ends of each leaf.

10. Divide filling mixture over each leaf evenly and fold in the sides.

11. Roll completely to enclose the filling.

12. Secure the rolls with toothpicks.

13. In the bottom of a baking dish, place 1/3 cup of tomato sauce evenly.

14. Arrange the rolls over sauce in a single layer.

15. Top with remaining sauce evenly.

16. Cover the baking dish and bake for about 15 minutes.

17. Remove from oven and immediately, sprinkle with the cheese.

18. Serve warm.

Nutrition Values (per serving)

Calories: 51

Fats: 6.5g

Carbs: 4.9g

Protein: 3.9g

Fiber: 1.9g

Lamb's Lettuce with Fresh Goat Cheese & Tomatoes

(Prepping time: 15 minutes| For 6 servings)

A healthy and delicious salad recipe… This salad is great for a light dinner. Lamb's lettuce and basil adds a delicious burst of garden fresh flavor to your salad plate.

Ingredients:

1 garlic clove, minced
3 tablespoons of extra-virgin olive oil
1 tablespoon of balsamic vinegar
Salt and freshly ground black pepper, to taste
2 pound of heirloom tomatoes, cored and cut into ½-inch thick wedges
2 tablespoons of fresh basil leaves, chopped
8 cups of lamb's lettuce, torn
1½-ounce of fresh goat cheese, crumbled
1/3 cup of small basil leaves

Preparation:

1. In a large bowl, add garlic, oil, vinegar, salt, and black pepper and beat until well combined.

2. Add tomato wedges and chopped basil and toss to combine.

3. Cover the bowl and keep at room temperature for about 1 hour, tossing occasionally.

4. On 6 serving plates, divide the lettuce evenly.

5. Place tomato mixture over lettuce evenly.

6. Top with goat cheese and basil leaves and serve.

Nutrition Values (per serving)

Calories: 131

Fats: 10g

Carbs: 8.5g

Protein: 3.9g

Fiber: 2.3g

Healthy Green Spiral Salad with Exotic Sea Weed

(Prepping time: 15 minutes | For 4 servings)

A fresh, tangy and crunchy veggie noodle salad with seaweed… This veggie noodle salad makes a really flavorful meal.

Ingredients:

For Salad:

2 zucchinis, spiralized with blade C
2 cucumbers, peeled and spiralized with blade C
¼ cup of wakame, soaked for about 10 minutes and drained
¼ cup of scallion, chopped

For Dressing:

½ teaspoon of fresh ginger, minced
1 garlic clove, minced
1½ tablespoons of extra-virgin olive oil
½ teaspoon of coconut aminos
1/8 teaspoon of red pepper flakes, crushed

Preparation:

1. Prepare the salad in a large bowl by mixing together all the ingredients except the scallions.

2. In another bowl, add all the dressing ingredients and beat until well combined.

3. Pour dressing over salad and toss to coat well.

4. Garnish with scallions and serve.

Nutrition Values (per serving)

Calories: 98

Fats: 5.8g

Carbs: 9.88g

Protein: 3g

Fiber: 2.3g

Papaya Pasta with Tasty & Spicy Dressing

(Prepping time: 15 minutes| For 6 servings)

A unique salad platter for your dinner table… Spicy dressing adds subtle flavors in a papaya noodle salad. This salad will be a great and delicious addition to your salad menu list.

Ingredients:

For Dressing:

> 2 garlic cloves, peeled
> 1 Serrano pepper, chopped
> 1 tablespoon of peanuts, toasted
> 1 teaspoons of powdered stevia
> Salt, to taste
> 2 tablespoons of fresh lime juice
> 1 teaspoon of coconut aminos

For salad:

> 2 papayas, peeled, seeded and spiralized with blade C
> 2 cups of grape tomatoes, quartered

Preparation:

1. Prepare the dressing in a blender by adding all the dressing ingredients and pulse until a paste forms.

2. Prepare the salad in a large bowl, mix together papaya noodles and tomatoes.

3. Pour dressing over salad and gently, toss to coat well.

Nutrition Values (per serving)

Calories: 68

Fats: 1.2g

Carbs: 14.8g

Protein: 1.6g

Fiber: 2.8g

Delightful Mixed Vegetable Noodles Salad with Exotic Sea Weeds

(Prepping time: 20 minutes| For 6 servings)

One of the best and nutritiously healthy salad… Arame seaweed and mixed veggie noodles make a wonderful combo. This simple dressing enhances the flavor of both the veggies and seaweed.

Ingredients:

- 2 medium zucchinis, spiralized with blade C
- 2 medium cucumbers, peeled and spiralized with blade C
- 2 medium carrots, peeled and spiralized with blade C
- 1 cup of dried arame seaweed, soaked for 15 minutes and drained
- 1 garlic clove, minced
- 2 tablespoons of extra-virgin olive oil
- 2 tablespoons of balsamic vinegar
- 1 teaspoon of coconut aminos

Preparation:

1. In a large bowl, add all the ingredients and toss to coat well.

2. Serve immediately.

Nutrition Values (per serving)

Calories: 94

Fats: 4.9g

Carbs: 12.1g

Protein: 1.7g

Fiber: 1.7g

Brilliant Red Noodles in Exotic Mushroom Sauce

(Prepping time: 15 minutes| Cooking time: 10 minutes| For 4 servings)

A true comforting food for your dinner table… This luscious creamy mushroom sauce gives a rich favor to healthy carrots. Even picky eaters will love to eat this meal.

Ingredients:

For Mushroom Sauce:

> 2 tablespoons of butter
> 2 garlic cloves, minced
> 1 tablespoon of fresh sage leaves, chopped
> 6-ounce of fresh Pprtobello mushrooms, sliced
> Salt and freshly ground black pepper, to taste
> ¼ cup of heavy cream
> 1 scallion, chopped

For Red Noodles:

> 3 large carrots, spiralized with blade C

Preparation:

1. In a large skillet, melt butter on medium heat.

2. Add garlic and basil and sauté for about 1 minute.

3. Add mushrooms, salt, and black pepper and cook 6-7 minutes.

4. Stir in heavy cream cook for about 1-2 minute.

5. Stir in scallions and remove from heat.

6. Divide the carrot noodles onto serving plates. Top with mushroom sauce evenly.

Nutrition Values (per serving)

Calories: 113

Fats: 8.7g

Carbs: 8g

Protein: 2.2g

Fiber: 2.1g

Tomato Magic with a Cheese Twist

(Prepping time: 10 minutes| For 6 servings)

A classic combination of tomatoes, fresh mozzarella, and basil… Balsamic vinegar adds a delicious tangy touch to this platter. This meal will be great for summer meals.

Ingredients:

3 large tomatoes, sliced
8-ounce of small fresh mozzarella cheese balls
¼ cup of balsamic vinegar
¼ cup of extra-virgin olive oil
Salt and freshly ground black pepper, to taste
¼ cup of fresh basil leaves, minced

Preparation:

1. On a large serving platter, arrange the tomato slices and mozzarella cheese balls.

2. In a bowl, add the vinegar, oil, salt, and black pepper and beat until well combined.

3. Drizzle the vinaigrette over the salad.

4. Top with basil and serve.

Nutrition Values (per serving)

Calories: 197

Fats: 15.3g

Carbs: 5g

Protein: 11.5g

Fiber: 1.1g

Garlic Grilled Zucchini

(Prepping time: 15 minutes| Cooking time: 4 minutes| For 4 servings)

One of the easiest and best recipes for a tasty zucchini… Grilling gives the zucchini a wonderful perfection of smoky flavors. Coating of garlic, Italian seasoning, butter, and lemon gives the zucchini a classic taste.

Ingredients:

4 garlic cloves, minced
¼ cup of unsalted butter, melted
2 tablespoons of fresh lemon juice
1 teaspoon of Italian seasoning
Salt and freshly ground black pepper, to taste
2 medium zucchinis, cut into ½-inch thick slices diagonally
2 tablespoons of fresh parsley leaves, minced

Preparation:

1. Preheat the grill to medium-high heat. Grease the grill grate with oil.

2. In a large bowl, mix together garlic, butter, lemon juice, Italian seasoning, salt, and black pepper.

3. Add zucchini slices and coat with garlic mixture generously.

4. Arrange the zucchini slices over grill in a single layer.

5. Grill for about 2 minutes per side.

6. Garnish with parsley and serve hot.

Nutrition Values (per serving)

Calories: 128

Fats: 12.1g

Carbs: 4.7g

Protein: 1.6g

Fiber: 1.2g

Peppers with Cheesy Vegetable Stuffing

(Prepping time: 20 minutes| Cooking time: 16 minutes| For 6 servings)

A restaurant-style stuffed bell peppers recipe that can be prepared easily at home… Surely you would love to make these stuffed peppers again and again.

Ingredients:

1 tablespoon of coconut oil
1 garlic clove, minced
1 cup of onion, chopped
1 pound of fresh mushrooms, chopped
½ tablespoon of red chili powder
½ tablespoon of ground cumin
Salt, to taste
½ cup of tomato puree
3 medium bell peppers, halved lengthwise and cored
1 cup of water
4-ounce of sharp cheddar cheese, shredded

Preparation:

1. In a skillet, melt coconut oil over medium-high heat.

2. Add garlic clove and sauté for about 1 minute

3. Add onions and mushrooms and cook for about 5-6 minutes.

4. Stir in spices and cook for about 1 minute.

5. Remove from heat and stir in tomato puree.

6. Meanwhile in a microwave-safe baking dish, arrange the bell peppers, cut-side down.

7. Pour water in baking dish.

8. With a plastic wrap, cover the baking dish and microwave on High for about 4-5 minutes.

9. Remove from microwave and uncover the baking dish.

10. Dain the water completely.

11. Now in the baking dish, arrange the bell peppers cut-side up.

12. Stuff the bell peppers with mushroom mixture evenly and top with cheese.

14. Microwave on high for about 2-3 minutes.

Nutrition Values (per serving)

Calories: 151

Fats: 9.2g

Carbs: 7.6g

Protein: 8.4g

Fiber: 2.7g

Chapter 5: Top Snack Recipes

Power Booster Cookies for Keto Dieters

(Prepping time: 15 minutes| Cooking time: 12 minutes| For 6 servings)

A simple recipe of delicious cookies… These cookies are best for those who likes to have a crispy treat with their coffee or tea… But, your kids will also love to enjoy these cookies.

Ingredients:

2 large organic eggs
1¼ cups of almond butter
1/3 cup of powdered erythritol
2/3 cup of unsweetened cacao powder
Salt, to taste

Preparation:

1. Preheat the oven to 320 degrees F. Line a large cookie sheet with parchment paper.

2. In a food processor, add all the ingredients and pulse until a dough forms.

3. Divide the dough into 12 equal sized balls.

4. Arrange the balls onto a prepared cookie sheet in a single layer.

5. With a fork, press down each ball into ½-inch thickness.

6. Bake for about 12 minutes. Serve warm.

Nutrition Values (per serving)

Calories: 66

Fats: 8.8g

Carbs: 5.8g

Protein: 4.7g

Fiber: 3.5g

Cashew Milk Smoothie with a Punch of Fruit

(Prepping time: 10 minutes| For 2 servings)

One of the best smoothie recipes with super healthy ingredients… Blueberries, cashew milk, and chia seeds make a healthy combo. The cashew milk adds a silky and creamy touch in this smoothie.

Ingredients:

- 1 cup of frozen blueberries
- 1½ cups of unsweetened cashew milk
- 1 tablespoon of chia seeds
- 3-4 drops of liquid stevia

Preparation:

1. In a high speed blender, add all the ingredients and pulse until smooth.
2. Pour into 2 serving glasses and serve immediately.

Nutrition Values (per serving)

Calories: 77

Fats: 6.48g

Carbs: 3g

Protein: 1.35g

Fiber: 3.55g

Bliss-of-Summer Watermelon Cooler

(Prepping time: 10 minutes| For 4 servings)

One of the easiest summer snacks to prepare... This watermelon cooler is just perfect for hot summer days. Watermelon, lime juice, stevia, and ice are simply blended together in this quick treat.

Ingredients:

4 cups of seedless watermelon, chopped
¼ cup of fresh lime juice
1 teaspoon of powdered stevia
Pinch of salt
Ice cubes, as required

Preparation:

1. In a high speed blender, add all the ingredients and pulse until smooth.
2. Pour into 4 serving glasses and serve immediately.

Nutrition Values (per serving)

Calories: 49

Fats: 0.2g

Carbs: 12.7g

Protein: 0.9g

Fiber: 0.7g

Chocolate & Strawberry Pancake

(Prepping time: 15 minutes\ Cooking time: 40 minutes |For 8 servings)

One of the best recipes for delicious pancakes… This sweet treat will be loved by adults and kids as well… These chocolaty strawberry pancakes have a light and fluffy texture.

Ingredients:

1¾ cups of almond flour
¼ teaspoon of baking soda
1/8 teaspoon of ground cinnamon
¾ cup of unsweetened almond milk
2 organic eggs
4-5 drops of liquid stevia
1/3 cup of fresh strawberries, hulled and sliced
¼ cup of mini unsweetened dark chocolate chips
2 tablespoons of olive oil

Preparation:

1. In a bowl, mix together flour, baking soda, and cinnamon.

2. In another bowl, add milk, eggs, and stevia and beat until well combined.

3. Add egg mixture into flour mixture and mix until well combined.

4. Fold in strawberries and chocolate chips.

5. Keep aside the mixture for about 5 minutes.

6. In a skillet, heat a little amount of oil on medium-high heat.

7. Add about 3 tablespoons of mixture in the skillet.

8. Cook for about 2-3 minutes.

9. Carefully, flip the pancake and cook for about 2 minutes more.

10. Repeat with the remaining oil and mixture.

Nutrition Values (per serving)

Calories: 200

Fats: 16.9g

Carbs: 8.3g

Protein: 6.3g

Fiber: 3g

Homemade Tomato Soup

(Prepping time: 20 minutes |For 8 servings)

An excellent way to enjoy fresh tomatoes in a cold soup… This soup is a delicious combo of tomatoes, veggies, lemon juice and vinegar. Definitely you would entertain your family with this satisfying and delicious cold soup.

Ingredients:

    4 large tomatoes, chopped
    1 large cucumber, peeled, seeded and chopped
    2/3 cup of red onion, chopped
    2 celery stalks, chopped
    3 garlic cloves, chopped
    2 tablespoons of balsamic vinegar
    2 tablespoons of fresh lemon juice
    Salt and freshly ground black pepper, to taste
    2 cups of vegetable broth
    ¼ cup of olive oil

Preparation:

1. In a blender, add all the ingredients except the olive oil and pulse until smooth.

2. While motor is running slowly, add the olive oil and pulse until smooth.

3. Serve immediately.

Nutrition Values (per serving)

Calories: 94

Fats: 6.9g

Carbs: 6.6g

Protein: 2.5g

Fiber: 1.6g

Ginger Peach Smoothie

(Prepping time: 10 minutes |For 2 servings)

One of the most super-versatile smoothies… Peaches, ginger, stevia, and coconut milk whip up into creamy, delicious smoothies in just minutes. Fresh ginger adds a healthy boosting touch in this smoothie.

Ingredients:

1 cup of frozen peaches, pitted and chopped
2 teaspoons of fresh ginger, chopped
5-6 drops of liquid stevia
¾ cup of unsweetened coconut milk

Preparation:

1. In a blender, add all ingredients and pulse until smooth.

2. Serve immediately.

Nutrition Values (per serving)

Calories: 243

Fats: 21.8g

Carbs: 13.3g

Protein: 2.9g

Fiber: 3.4g

Super Healthy Beet Greens Salad

(Prepping time: 10 minutes |For 4 servings)

An easy salad with simple ingredients… These beet greens make a really refreshing salad for you.

Ingredients:

For Dressing:

- 1 garlic clove, minced
- 1 ½ teaspoons of dijon mustard
- 3 tablespoons of extra-virgin olive oil
- 1 tablespoon balsamic vinegar
- Salt and freshly ground black pepper, to taste
- 2 cups of vegetable broth
- ¼ cup of olive oil

For Salad:

- 8 cup of fresh beet greens
- ¼ cup of feta cheese, crumbled

Preparation:

1. Prepare dressing in a bowl by adding all the dressing ingredients and beat until well combined.

2. In a large bowl, mix together greens and cheese.

3. Pour dressing over salad and toss to coat well. Serve immediately.

<u>Nutrition Values (per serving)</u>

Calories: 280

Fats: 26.2g

Carbs: 9.1g

Protein: 5.5g

Fiber: 3.6g

Coconut Yogurt with Chia Seeds and Almonds

(Prepping time: 10 minutes |For 4 servings)

A healthy and wonderfully delicious treat for the whole family… This delicious treat needs no cooking. Chia seeds, almond milk, and coconut yogurt marry each other nicely.

Ingredients:

For Dressing:

> 1 1/3 cups of coconut yogurt
> 1 cup of unsweetened almond milk
> 8-10 drops of liquid stevia
> Pinch of salt
> 1/3 cup of chia seeds
> 3 tablespoons of almonds, chopped

Preparation:

1. In a bowl, add yogurt, milk, stevia, and salt and beat until well combined.

2. Add chia seeds and beat until well combined.

3. Refrigerate, covered for at least 4 hours.

4. Serve with a sprinkle of chopped almonds.

Nutrition Values (per serving)

Calories: 182

Fats: 9.1g

Carbs: 14.4g

Protein: 4.7g

Fiber: 10.8g

Super Delicious Cucumber Salad

(Prepping time: 10 minutes |For 8 servings)

A refreshing and creamy salad with the crunchiness of fresh cucumbers... this fresh salad is great for cucumber lovers. Cream, vinegar, stevia, and dill weed adds a really delicious flavoring to cucumbers.

Ingredients:

½ cup of sour cream
1 teaspoon of white vinegar
½ teaspoon of powdered stevia
½ teaspoon of dill weed
Salt, to taste
4 medium cucumbers, sliced

Preparation:

1. In a bowl, add all the ingredients except cucumbers and beat until well combined.

2. Add cucumber slices and stir until well combined.

3. Refrigerate to chill for at least 30 minutes before serving.

Nutrition Values (per serving)

Calories: 54

Fats: 3.2g

Carbs: 6.1g

Protein: 1.4g

Fiber: 0.8g

Pudding Delight with Banana & Coconut

(Prepping time: 15 minutes |For 4 servings)

A really delicious sweet treat with the combo of banana, yogurt, coconut milk, and shredded coconut… The combination makes a really indulgent sweet treat for the whole family.

Ingredients:

- 1 medium banana, peeled and quartered
- 2 tablespoons of unsweetened coconut milk
- 1 packet of stevia
- 1 teaspoon of vanilla extract
- 1 cup of plain greek yogurt
- 2 tablespoons of unsweetened coconut, shredded

Preparation:

1. In a blender, add quartered bananas, milk, stevia, and vanilla extract and beat until well combined and smooth.

2. Transfer the mixture into a bowl.

3. Gently, fold in yogurt.

4. Refrigerate to chill completely.

5. Garnish with coconut and serve.

Nutrition Values (per serving)

Calories: 103

Fats: 4g

Carbs: 10.2g

Protein: 6.9g

Fiber: 1.2g

Extra Easy Cheese Sandwich

(Prepping time: 15 mins| Cooking time: 5 mins 40 seconds | For 1 serving)

A wonderful recipe for a cheese sandwich… These homemade sandwich really tastes like grilled cheese sandwiches.

Bun Ingredients:

    2 tablespoons of almond flour
    2 tablespoons of butter, softened
    1½ tablespoons of psyllium husk powder
    ½ teaspoon of baking powder
    2 large organic eggs

For Sandwiches:

    2 tablespoons of cheddar cheese, grated
    1 tablespoon of butter

Preparation:

1. In a bowl, add all the bun ingredients except eggs and mix until a dough forms.

2. Add eggs and mix until a thick dough forms.

3. Press each dough in a microwave safe square container.

5. Smooth the surface and clean of the sides.

6. Microwave for about 90-100 seconds.

7. Remove from microwave and keep aside to cool slightly.

8. Carefully remove the bun from container.

9. Cut the bun in half.

10. Place the cheese over cut side of 1 bun slices.

11. Cover with remaining bun slice to make a sandwich.

12. In a skillet, melt butter on medium heat.

13. Add sandwich and cook for about 1-2 minutes per side.

Nutrition Values (per serving)

Calories: 577

Fats: 55.1g

Carbs: 4.7g

Protein: 19g

Fiber: 1.6g

India Super Easy Summer Cooler

(Prepping time: 5 minutes| For 2 servings)

A chilled summer treat that is popular in all of India… This chilled yogurt cooler is really refreshing and light. Spices add a delicious kick in this chilled summer cooler.

Ingredients:

1 cup of plain greek yogurt
1 cup of chilled water
Pinch of ground cumin
Pinch of paprika
Pinch of salt

Preparation:

1. In a bowl, add yogurt and beat until smooth.
2. Slowly, add water, beating continuously.
3. Add spices and stir to combine well.
4. Pour into 2 serving glasses and serve immediately.

Nutrition Values (per serving)

Calories: 48

Fats: 1.3g

Carbs: 2.6g

Protein: 6.3g

Fiber: 0g

Conclusion

This book gives you healthy and scrumptious choices of foods to pick from to create 50 keto-friendly recipes. When you apply this diet to your day-to-day life, you will definitely achieve your expected results. These recipes are given with their nutritional values too, so you know exactly what you're eating. Restricting carbs and sugar with this diet will also control blood sugar levels in your body. This is a whole food diet that is free from processed or unhealthy junk foods. Once you get used to the healthy ingredients, you can then plan your own meals having keto-friendly foods. So heads up, eat healthy and become slimmer and stronger!

Made in the USA
Middletown, DE
28 December 2019